Off the Grid With the Kids

A Pediatricians Guide to Foreign Travel with your Children

Don LaGrone, MD, FAAP

Introduction: Why this book?

While anchored in an isolated cove on the west coast of Puerto Rico I encountered a family of six, planning to circumnavigate the globe. Of their four children, two less than six years of age had histories of asthma. The father approached me, as a physician, for advice regarding his 4-year-old who had been wheezing and short of breath for a week. They had only a small supply of rescue inhalers on board! He had nothing to use if the rescue inhaler failed! Fortunately, I was able to provide prescriptions for the medication their child needed, as well as additional supplies for their journey.

Many Americans avoid traveling "off the grid" with their children, due to fear of illness and the anticipation that medical resources will not be available. Some concerns are well founded, particularly for overland travel in very remote areas or for long ocean passages, where a higher degree of preparation and self-reliance are required. Likewise, children with chronic, relapsing, or unstable medical problems are at higher risk when distant from medical services. That being said, too many families with otherwise healthy children succumb to the concerns of well-meaning relatives and friends, canceling life-enhancing trips in the planning stage.

Independent foreign travel gives children a better understanding of the realities of life for the majority of our neighbors, providing an enriched context for decisions they will make as adults. Leaving the tourists behind requires commitment, but the rewards are substantial. Viewing giraffes at DisneyWorld or the local zoo simply does not compare with camping as a family on the Serengeti! A visit to SeaWorld is not the same as standing on the bow of your own boat hundreds or thousands of miles from land and watching dolphins frolic in your bow wave! But what if your child becomes ill, or is injured? In writing this book I will try to answer that question. No amount of preparation can completely remove all the risks associated with traveling "off the grid", but as you will see, most risks are small, or can be substantially mitigated by preparation. If you've considered travel "off the grid" and hesitated, read on.

Why me?

While in medical school I took much of the coursework for my master's degree in public health and tropical medicine, as well as performing externships in surgery in Salzburg, Austria, and internal medicine at Kings College Hospital, London. After completing my internship, my wife and 2-year-old son accompanied me to Botswana, where I served as the medical representative for U S Peace Corps operations in Southern Africa and ran a 75-bed tuberculosis hospital. During our 3 year stay, we traveled throughout southern Africa, enjoying numerous camping trips into the bush, with our son, often many miles from roads or centers of the local population. At the end of my tour of duty, we drove overland thousands of miles through Botswana, Zambia, Tanzania, Kenya, Malawi, and Zimbabwe before returning to the US. After completing my residency in Pediatrics, during which my daughter was born, we moved to Pago Pago, American Samoa - midway between Hawaii and New Zealand, where I spent two years as director of Pediatric services at the LBJ Tropical Medical Center. At the end of that tour, my family, with children now aged 3 and 9 years, crewed a friends 40 ft. sailboat from Papua New Guinea via Australia and the 7,000-mile Indian Ocean to Africa. After six months at sea, we returned to the US, where I practiced pediatrics for 30 years on the Gulf Coast of Mississippi. In 2008 I joined the rapid response team of Medical Teams International and participated in relief trips to Haiti and the Philippines in response to earthquakes, hurricanes and outbreaks of Cholera. In 2016 I retired, bought a sail-boat, and traveled with my wife through the Florida Keys, Bahamas, Dominican Republic, Puerto Rico and the Caribbean islands as far as Martinique. I continue to think as a Pediatrician, but with a background in "off the grid" international travel. While I am not an expert in every aspect of Medicine, I bring a unique perspective to the subject of foreign travel with children, which I hope will help inform you in your own decisions as you plan your adventures - Off the Grid with your children.

Table of Contents

Topic	Page
General considerations - travel with children	1
Immunizations	2
Drinking water and food abroad	3-4
History of Past Medical Problems	5
Medical Providers Abroad	5-6
Communications when Off the Grid	7-12
Medical Evacuation	13
Fever	14
Non-specific Febrile Illness	16
Gastroenteritis	17
Dehydration	19
Secretory Diarrhea	20

Dysentery	21
Colitis	22
Typhoid Fever	23
Abdominal Pain	24
Jaundice	25
Pharyngitis (sore throat)	27
Otitis (ear ache)	27
Nosebleeds	28
Cough	29
Croup	30
Pneumonia	31
Asthma	32
Systemic Allergic Reactions	33
Insect Bites	34
Skin and Soft Tissue Infections	36

Abscess	38
Fungal Skin Infections	38
Lacerations	39
Puncture Wounds	40
Fish Hook Removal	41
Burns	42-43
Head Injury	44
Seizures	45
Dislocations	47-50
Fractures	52
Urinary Tract Infection	53
Vulvovaginitis	55

Regional Considerations

North Australia and SW Pacific		56
Temperate Australia and New Zealand		57
South Asia		63
Africa		67

Appendix I   Pediatric Drugs and Doses   70-81

Appendix II   Information Sources   82

Appendix III   Medical Evacuation   83

Travel with Children: General Considerations;

A great deal of foreign travel does not necessitate any health planning. Urban centers throughout the world have up-to-date medical facilities, and qualified providers and have controlled the vectors of transmissible diseases. In this respect, London is little different from New York!

Traveling in rural areas or may require awareness of the location of healthcare facilities, but that is not what I intend by "off the grid". The intrepid traveler who leaves the paved roads behind and heads into the bush, or sails across open ocean passages has truly gone "off the grid", and must consider the risks as well as the benefits involved.

Many aspects of health we take for granted at home, such as the availability of fresh safe food and water, exposure to unusual illnesses, and the potential separation from health services need to be taken into account when planning your trip. That being said, after years of travel and residence in Africa and the South Pacific, I look back at those times as some of the healthiest in our lives. Western schools and childcare facilities are breeding grounds for the viral infections which so often affect our children. On board a sailboat or overland vehicle exposure to other children is greatly reduced, as is the risk of common illnesses. On the other hand, diseases such as polio, and measles, which are highly contagious, still exist in some countries, although properly immunized children are well protected. Exotic tropical diseases such as malaria can be avoided through the use of prophylactic medication.

Immunizations:

The availability of safe and effective vaccines for many of the childhood illnesses that contributed to high mortality in previous centuries has been the greatest breakthrough in Pediatrics. All children without a medical contraindication should receive ALL of the available vaccinations. The organisms which cause diphtheria, whooping cough, tetanus, polio, measles, meningitis, pneumonia, hepatitis A &B, and influenza STILL EXIST - in the United States and around the world. The ONLY reason most of these diseases have become rare at home is that nearly all children are immunized. Unimmunized children are at high risk of becoming ill when exposed, and exposure is more likely when you travel abroad. Children who have not received all recommended immunizations should not travel!

Additional immunizations for yellow fever, typhoid, and cholera may be indicated in some areas of travel. Likewise, prophylaxis against malaria may be appropriate in certain seasons and regions of some countries. For information on the currently recommended vaccinations or prophylaxis for your planned area of travel, consult the guidelines at: wwwnc.cdc.gov/travel, or discuss with your physician.

2

Drinking Water:

Most areas of the world have safe drinking water in urban centers. Rural water supplies are less reliable and should be avoided. A safe guideline for boaters and others who carry a supply of water with them is to fill tanks with water from a reverse osmosis system. If not available, local tap water can be treated by adding plain unscented bleach in a ratio of 2 teaspoons bleach per 10 gallons of water. Allow to stand for one hour prior to use. Always use RO or treated water to

wash fresh fruits and vegetables and make ice. Excellent filters are available from outdoor supply stores, which eliminate bacteria and protozoa from water, making it safe to drink.

The quantity of water available is equally important. Under normal conditions, the average adult member of your party will need about 1 liter of drinking water per day. Those working in hot conditions may require up to 16 liters per day. Children aged 4-8 years need a total of 7-10 cups of water per day - under normal conditions. Older children and teens need 10-15 cups/day, including water found in foods and soft drinks. Assuring an adequate supply of safe water should be part of your planning.

Food:

It would be a terrible shame to pass up mangos and other exotic fruits and vegetables during a trip due to fear of diarrhea! Any fruit that is peeled prior to eating (ie mangos, pineapple, and citrus) does not represent a hazard. Enjoy them. Lettuce, tomatoes, sprouts, and other leafy veggies which are neither cooked nor peeled represent a higher risk and should be washed with treated water prior to consumption. Salads and other dishes offered in roadside eateries are best avoided since whether precautions were taken in their preparation is unknown. Meats are generally safe if cooked thoroughly. Fish are generally safe, with the exception of Pelagic fish, such as tuna, swordfish, and marlin which carry a risk of mercury poisoning and should be eaten sparingly. Most authorities suggest one meal weekly. Likewise, in tropical waters ciguatera toxin accumulates in the flesh of carnivorous fish that feed around coral reefs. There is no test for ciguatera, and though local mythology may suggest means of determining if a given fish is affected, large predatory fish such as cubera snapper and large barracuda probably carry the greatest risk. If locals avoid a given fish, you'd be wise to follow suit. Since your supply of fresh fruits and vegetables may be inconsistent, a daily multivitamin is a good precaution during extended travel.

History of Past Medical Problems:

Children who have been healthy, aside from occasional colds or loose stools, should have not problems off the grid. With certain brief exceptions, my family's general health, while traveling through rural Africa or on extended sails, has been excellent. On the other hand, children with chronic or unstable medical conditions represent a much higher level of risk when medical support may be days away. For example, a child with type 1 (insulin-dependent) diabetes, who requires a ready supply of refrigerated insulin may experience complications during acute illnesses. Likewise, a child with an unstable or poorly controlled seizure disorder, or severe asthma is at greater risk. In my professional opinion, taking such children "off the grid" represents an unacceptable risk, for themselves and their parents.

Medical providers abroad;

In all but the most remote locations, local populations have some level of medical support, be that a rural nurse, village clinic, or local hospital. Many of the doctors one might encounter were trained in Europe or the United States. Facilities vary in complexity, hygiene, and resources. On the other hand, local practitioners are well versed in the diagnosis and treatment of illnesses that are common in their area. By comparison, an excellently trained emergency room physician in Cleveland, Ohio would be unlikely to consider or recognize dengue fever or malaria as the cause of a febrile illness! In general, I believe you may (and often must) rely on your own ability to diagnose and treat simple illnesses and injuries. In cases where this is not sufficient, reliance on local medical professionals is the next step. Only in rare, complicated or prolonged illnesses should evacuation be necessary.

<u>Pharmacies:</u>

In many countries, you may purchase medications at a local pharmacy that would require a prescription at home. In appendix 1 I have listed useful medications under their generic names, as well as trade names you might recognize. I have also included available dosage forms best suited for traveling children and the appropriate dose and dosage intervals. If you will be traveling far from support, your medical provider should be willing to assist you with prescriptions for the drugs you wish to carry with you, prior to your departure. I recommend that you carry a durable supply of the drugs you feel you might need, including medications for any chronic or recurring illness such as asthma and high-frequency conditions such as fever, simple infections, and diarrhea. Other medicines may be purchased from local pharmacies abroad. When requesting a medication from a foreign pharmacy, always use the generic name, which the pharmacist is more likely to recognize, (ie. ask for acetaminophen, not Tylenol).

Communications:

Modern world travelers have access to advanced communications technologies. Cell phones, many of which contain GPS chips, have become common in underdeveloped countries. Reception maps should be compared to your travel plans. You will either need an international roaming program from your home country's cellular provider or a "SIM card" from a local cellular provider. Not all smartphones allow you to change the sim card. Some are "locked" by the provider. Check before you travel, to see that your phone is "unlocked" and can accept a new sim card. Cell phones allow voice, data, and voice over internet communications. With a local data plan, you can use programs such as WhatsApp, Skype, or FaceTime to stay in touch with family and friends at home, as long as you have cell reception. You may also be able to call your child's physician from abroad. Be sure you have their contact details.

What about communications at sea or in areas where no cell connection is possible? At the time of writing, satellite telephones remain expensive, but allow virtually worldwide communication. Satellite position locators are more affordable and allow travelers to text messages worldwide. In the event of an emergency, the SOS function will put you in touch with resources for evacuation and allow continuous contact until help arrives.

Whether you are trekking across the Kalahari Desert in Botswana or sailing the high seas, impor tant choices relate to how FAR off the grid you are willing to be! If a medical emergency or mechanical breakdown occurs, how well can you cope on your own? When you are hundreds of miles from civilization, it can take days to get in touch, and even longer for help to arrive.

Technology now allows rapid communication with emergency responders. In general, the cost varies directly with the level of connectivity. Available resources are changing so rapidly that it is impossible to list all the available technology and costs, but I will try to give you a representative sample of what is current as of the publication date.

Single Side Band Radio

This is an older technology, used primarily on ships at sea, that relies on signals bounced off the stratosphere for long-distance communication. SSB reception is dependent on atmospheric conditions, which vary daily, and seasonally. It is also affected by solar flares, weather, and other atmospheric conditions, making reception unreliable. The learning curve needed to use the equipment is steep. SSB radios are more expensive than modern Satellite phones, less reliable, and much more difficult to use. I mention them for completeness only and would not recommend investing in this technology.

Satellite Communicators

The earth is surrounded by a maze of commercial and military satellites that allow continuous monitoring of your position as well as supporting different forms of communication. The Iridium Satellite Network has 66 low earth orbit satellites, providing virtually complete coverage of the globe. Three levels of satellite communication are available.

EPIRB Units (emergency position indicating radio beacon)

This technology has been available since the 1970s. When activated the beacon, which contains a GPS receiver and is preprogrammed with information identifying the user, transmits radio frequency signals at two frequencies that are picked up by satellites and aircraft and subsequently transmitted to responding agencies. They are not strictly speaking communicators, since they cannot transmit voice or text messages. Also, the unit must be registered and deployed or activated to be useful. They are primarily used by boaters. A small handheld example is the ACR Res-QLink 400, which costs about $300, and does not require a subscription. Since there is no transmit function, it is limited to providing an SOS signal and your location.

GPS-based satellite messengers

This mid-level device has become very popular with off-the-grid travelers and is equally useful on land or sea. Like the EPIRB the owner's information is registered with a 24/7 worldwide monitoring service that tracks your location via the iridium satellite system every few minutes. This allows friends and family at home to follow your travels in real-time on a computer. Each unit has an SOS function, actuated by a protected switch, which transmits your location and identifying information to an emergency response monitor. These units have the capacity to send and receive text messages, so you are able to explain to the monitoring agency exactly the nature and urgency of your problem. It likewise allows continuous communication until the problem is resolved, or help arrives. Examples include:

Garmin In Reach Satellite Messenger

This sturdy pocket-sized unit costs about $450. It requires a $20 activation fee and monthly subscription, varying from $12 to $80 based on the number of text messages desired, availability of marine and weather forecasts, etc. They use the global iridium satellite system, are rechargeable, and highly reliable.

Spot X Explorer Satellite Messenger

Similar to the In Reach, this unit costs about $230. It has a $25 annual fee and a $12 - 40/month subscription fee based on the number of text messages allowed. The Spot X replaced a previous model which only allowed preprogrammed messages and at the time of writing its reviews have been mixed.

Iridium Go Satellite Hotspot

Coupled with a smartphone (Apple or Android) this $795 unit converts your cell phone to a satellite phone, allowing voice calling and text messaging as well as enhanced data capabilities for email and weather monitoring. It also offers a 100 ft. radius Wi-Fi connection for up to 5 mobile devices. A 50-minute voice subscription costs $139/month after a $50 activation fee. Data calls and text messages are unlimited. The unit does not have an automated SOS function.

Satellite Telephones

These represent the highest level of communication and demand the highest price. With a Sat-Phone, you can pick up the handset and call anywhere in the world, from anywhere in the world, at any time. The system isn't perfect and areas of decreased reception may occur. Likewise, atmospheric conditions may occasionally limit reception, but they are far more reliable than the SSB Radio. Numerous equipment and service providers exist. A current internet search yielded the following:

Iridium handset from $627

Globalstar handset from $500

Inmarsat handset from $600

Each phone requires a monthly service plan, whose cost is based on the amount of "talk time" used. For example, Iridium charges the following monthly subscription rates: 20 minutes/mo. $60

40 minutes/mo.	$75
60 minutes/mo	$10
200 minutes/mo	$240

Combined with a GPS for location information, these units offer the most rapid and complete ability to communicate from the bush or at sea. Unlike satellite messengers and SSB radio, they do not have a push-button SOS function that automatically identifies you and your location.

Evacuation

In the event that you should require immediate emergency assistance or evacuation - your sailboat is sinking, or your child is severely ill or injured while remote from aid, three intervals separate you from safety. The first is the time necessary to call for help. Depending on your location this could take days without a satellite communicator. Once your SOS is received and your location acquired, contact will be made with the closest governmental or commercial resource to be mobilized. Depending on your location that could be local police, ambulance, military, coast guard, navy, ships at sea, etc. Once you have contacted an SOS responder, they will require time to organize resources and reach your location. Again, the delay will be directly proportional to the remoteness of your location. The third delay involves returning you to safety. Clearly, the more remote your travels, the greater the self-reliance needed. After all, that's why yachts have life rafts! No one expects to cross the ocean in a raft, but for the hours or days before rescue, it certainly beats treading water. Since the safety of others may be jeopardized by your evacuation, such requests should be made ONLY in life-threatening emergencies.

Your evacuation and your treatment abroad may also generate significant financial exposure. This is magnified if your condition warrants an emergent return to your home country. Even though the likelihood of evacuation is small, insurance is available to protect you from the financial consequences. Appendix 3 lists some of the currently available resources to defray the expense of foreign medical evacuation and treatment.

Fever:

It is important to recognize that fever in itself is harmless. Our bodies create the elevation in temperature we recognize as fever, in response to chemical mediators of inflammation released by our white blood cells. This is part of our immune response, most often in response to infection. It is these mediators that cause fever, as well as the aches and pains that encourage us to curl up in bed, saving our energy for dealing with the infection.

Since ancient times people have associated an elevated temperature with poor outcomes, such as death or brain damage. Since our ancestors did not know the cause of illnesses, they blamed poor outcomes on the one thing they could recognize, the fever. Fever gets our attention, and provides a useful measure of improvement, but should not remain the focus of your attention. The vast majority of childhood fevers are caused by simple viral infections which require no specific treatment on your part and resolve spontaneously.

The "normal" range of temperature for children in good health is from 97 to 100.8 degrees Fahrenheit (36.1 - 38.2 degrees Celsius). A low fever is a temperature of 101-102 degrees F, (38.3 - 38.9 C). Higher fevers of 103-104 F, (39.4-40 C) also occur with benign virus infections and are not dangerous. You may elect to treat the fever, but always LOOK BEYOND the fever for symptoms of the underlying illness.

The sudden onset of fever may precipitate a benign Febrile Seizure in young children. Such brief (<5 minutes) convulsions are frightening to bystanders but are not dangerous. Although some youngsters appear prone to febrile seizures before 4 years of age, their occurrence does not presage later seizures in the absence of fever. Fever increases the body's water consumption. Otherwise, no amount of the fever is dangerous. I have treated children with temperatures of 106-108 degrees F, without findings of serious illness, with observation and simple supportive measures such as acetaminophen (Tylenol) and fluids, until the fever abated. All recovered uneventfully, without antibiotics!

Strictly speaking, it is not necessary to treat fever, which often provides a useful gauge of the resolution of the underlying illness. Nonetheless, temperatures higher than 102 degrees Fahrenheit leave us feeling miserable, do not appear to assist the immune response, and may be treated on a compassionate basis.

The safest and most effective medication for fever and pain in children is acetaminophen (Tylenol). The dosage for children based upon their weight is equal to 10mg per kilogram of body weight and may be repeated at intervals of 4-6 hours. Such a calculation is more accurate than doses based on a range of weights.

Liquid Tylenol is available as 160mg per 5ml. syrup as well as chewable tablets. Use a syringe or measure, not a "teaspoon" which may vary in volume. Tylenol is remarkably safe, having a very wide range between effective and toxic dosages. You should take care that any OTHER medicines you are using do not also contain acetaminophen.

If you decide to treat fever, always wait at least 30 minutes after giving acetaminophen before applying cooling sponge baths. If you try to cool a child prior to Tylenol onset you may precipitate shivering, as the body attempts to maintain the elevated temperature through muscle contraction. NEVER sponge a child with alcohol, which can be absorbed through the skin and cause seizures.

Non-specific Febrile Illness

One of the most perplexing problems confronting a parent or physician is the child with fever and non-specific symptoms such as rash, myalgia (muscle pain), headache, and lethargy. The history may provide clues as to which illness is present. Exposure to mosquitoes suggests arbovirus infections, such as Zika, West Nile Fever, or Malaria. If tick bites are present typhus or rocky mt. spotted Fever are possible. In some locations, dengue fever, or malaria are possible. Lack of immunizations could raise the possibility of measles, or polio.

The most common infections producing non-specific symptoms are caused by viruses, for which there are no effective treatments, but which resolve spontaneously. In these cases assigning a specific diagnosis is of minimal practical value. Advanced laboratory tests would be needed and while they are pending only supportive care is indicated. Diagnosis is usually "retrospective", the child having improved or recovered before a diagnosis becomes available.

Rickettsial infections (Typhus, RMSF) or Leptospirosis may have similar symptoms but are more severe and prolonged. They all respond to Doxycycline. Malaria is unlikely unless prophylaxis has not been used during travel in a high-risk area.

When traveling "off the grid", without access to laboratory facilities, a reasonable approach to a prolonged febrile illness may involve treatment with Doxycycline to cover the treatable infections, if malaria is not in question. In underdeveloped countries where malaria is prevalent, febrile patients are often treated for malaria on presentation to the hospital, pending lab testing. In any case, continued observation and support will either provide reassurance that the illness is resolving or if the child's condition deteriorates, that emergency evacuation is necessary. I will return to this vexing quandary when we consider specific infections and regions of travel.

Gastroenteritis - vomiting and diarrhea

By far the most common illness encountered by travelers of any age is diarrhea, with or without fever and vomiting. Throughout the world, the majority (50-70%) of all cases of diarrhea are caused by virus infections, which are benign, mild, and limited to several days. Vomiting may limit fluid intake, while frequent watery stools greatly increase fluid losses. The risk of dehydration, particularly in children, becomes the primary concern. The vast majority of causes of diarrhea do not require specific therapy! That being said, diarrheal diseases represent the most frequent cause of death worldwide in children - due to dehydration.

Diarrhea

Diarrhea is present when a child has loose to watery stool that is more frequent than normal. This is caused by a combination of increased intestinal motility and the secretion of fluid into the intestine. Both mechanisms are usually operative during diarrhea, the reaction representing the body's attempt to "wash out" an offending pathogen. At its onset, diarrheal stools may be frequent, large in volume, and watery. This combination causes increased water loss from the body and contributes to the risk of dehydration. The first aspect of diarrhea to improve is usually the frequency of stooling, while the child continues to have large watery, but less frequent bowel movements. The second is the volume of stool. Thus the child continues to have watery stool, but it is less frequent and of smaller volume. It is quite common for children with benign cases of diarrhea to continue to have loose to watery stools for UP TO 2 WEEKS. If there is no blood or mucous in the stool, and neither fever nor abdominal pain, the persistence of loose stool is not a cause of concern!

Vomiting

Many cases of common diarrheal illness are associated with vomiting, particularly at the onset. Vomiting adds to the fluid losses caused by diarrhea and prevents the intake of replacement fluids. Fortunately, vomiting usually peaks early and resolves within 12 hours. Whenever vomiting and diarrhea coexist the risk of dehydration is increased!

Dehydration

I cannot overemphasize the importance of maintaining good hydration in this disease. Loses of water and salts must be replaced by drinking frequently, preferably an oral rehydration solution (ORS), containing salts, sugar, and water. Juices, soft drinks, and sports drinks contain excessive amounts of sugar and should be avoided. ORS is available on Amazon and in pharmacies as packets of flavored effervescent tablets (Hydralyte or Drip Drop) which are mixed with safe water. ORS is also widely available from rural clinics in underdeveloped countries. The approximate number of ounces needed over the first 4 hours of illness will equal a child's weight in pounds (ie a 40 lb. child will need 40 oz of ROS). Subsequent volumes depend on the amount of vomiting, the coexistence of fever, and the size and frequency of diarrheal stools. The patient should be encouraged to drink as much ORS as they wish. If vomiting is present, treatment with Ondansetron (Zofran), may be used (see appendix 1). In addition, giving smaller more frequent amounts of ORS may limit vomiting. As dehydration resolves urine output will increase and the color of the urine will become less dark.

Elevated temperatures (> 101 degrees F.) increase the water requirements of the body by 2.5 ml/kg/d for each degree above 98. Thus a 10kg child with a temperature of 102 degrees would have an increase in daily fluid requirement of 100 ml (a little over 3 oz.). When fever coexists with vomiting and diarrhea, the risk of dehydration is increased.

Signs of moderate dehydration include thirst, sunken eyes, dry mouth, and decreased production of dark urine. In severe dehydration lethargy, dry tongue, weak rapid pulses, low blood pressure, and absent urination occur. Gastroenteritis is the most common cause of death in children worldwide, due to dehydration! That it is not a serious problem in developed countries is due to the ready availability of medical intervention. When you travel "off the grid" YOU represent the first step in such intervention. Gastroenteritis with severe dehydration continues to represent a serious threat, averted by your early and intense response. Should that fail, seek help. For the purposes of this text I will divide diarrheal disease into three categories: secretory diarrhea, dysentery, and colitis, although overlap exists between them.

Secretory Diarrhea:

In this condition, the lining of the bowel secretes large amounts of watery fluid into the intestinal lumen. Blood is not present in the stool and fever is usually absent or mild. At the onset, vomiting may predominate, but this usually subsides within 12 hours as diarrhea continues. The most common cause of secretory diarrhea is infection with a virus or a strain of e.Coli bacteria (the classic "tourista"). Viral diarrhea usually resolves within 36 hours. Although e.Coli is the most common bacteria in the normal gut, some strains produce a toxin that causes diarrhea. The illness subsides in the vast majority of cases within 3-7 days. The only treatment required is hydration. Another less common, but much more severe cause of secretory diarrhea is Cholera. Infection with the cholera bacteria causes very severe rapid and profuse diarrhea. In fact, patients have been known to empty the serous component of their blood volume into the intestine so rapidly that they have gone into shock, before the passage of the first stool. Although untreated cholera is often fatal, antibiotic treatment is not necessary. Just as in e.Coli diarrhea, it is severe dehydration, not the infection itself that is dangerous.

As a general rule, although they may shorten the duration of diarrhea in secretory diarrhea, antibiotic medications are not needed for this condition. Bismuth subsalicylate (Pepto Bismol) may reduce diarrhea and is safe in children. Medicines that slow intestinal motility (Imodium and Lomotil) should be avoided as they inhibit the body"s need to shed the toxin, may prolong illness, and increase the risk of complications.

If diarrhea persists beyond 5-7 days and is associated with worsening dehydration, fever, or bloody stool, medical assistance should be sought. Prolonged diarrhea may also warrant the use of Azithromycin in younger children or Ciprofloxacin in teens or adults.

Dysentery

If acute diarrhea is associated with abdominal cramps, blood, and mucous-containing stool with substantial fever, the cause is more likely to be a strain of Shigella or a Shiga-toxin-producing e. Coli. As in secretory diarrhea, the primary approach to treatment is avoidance of dehydration by the use of ORS, although, in dysentery, the volume of stool is generally lower, making dehydration less likely. Although the bacteria that cause dysentery are susceptible to antibiotics, the majority of children do not require them. What's more, the use of an antibiotic in a child with

bloody diarrhea actually INCREASES the risk of complications, some of which can be fatal. Only in children with severe cramps, high fever, and lethargy, or in children less than 3 months of age should a course of antibiotics be initiated. In children, Azithromycin is the drug of choice, while Ciprofloxacin is used in teens and adults. Anti-motility agents such as loperamide (Imodium) or diphenoxylate (Lomotil) should be avoided, as they increase the risk of complications and may prolong the illness.

If available, a stool culture should precede the use of antibiotics, to identify the cause and local susceptibility of the organism. If a child has a bloody stool with a high fever and dehydration not resolving on ORS treatment, you should seek local medical support. The absence of urine output despite adequate hydration warrants immediate evacuation.

Colitis

Cases of infectious colitis have a more indolent onset, with fever, abdominal cramps, and blood or mucous in the stool, but rarely substantial diarrhea. Numerous causes include amoebic, bacterial, and parasite infections. Although dehydration is seldom a risk, empiric therapy is complicated by the need for a specific diagnosis. Stool specimens should be provided to a local facility to guide treatment. Fortunately, this presentation allows more time. The overlap between these three categories of illness can make diagnosis difficult. Supportive treatment with ORS and acetaminophen is indicated for all. Should the child develop bloody diarrhea associated with high fever and lethargy, or fail to resolve within 5-7 days, treatment with appropriate antibiotics should be given. When available, a stool culture is helpful.

<u>Typhoid fever</u>

Enteric fever (typhoid) is caused by infection with a strain of Salmonella bacteria, usually acquired from contaminated food or water. Illness presents with abdominal pain, diarrhea, fever, and chills, 1-3 weeks after infection. Fever normally increases the heart rate, yet children with enteric fever tend to have a slow pulse. A rash may be present on the trunk which is classically described as flat salmon-colored patches. Enteric fever should be suspected in a child with fever and GI symptoms of more than 3 days duration, who has traveled in an endemic area. Definitive diagnosis requires cultures not available "off the grid". Untreated enteric fever may be complicated by intestinal perforation, systemic bacterial infection, and death. For this reason, presumptive therapy is appropriate. The drug of choice for children is Azithromycin is used once daily for 7 days. Ciprofloxacin is a reasonable alternative if Azithromycin is not available, but resistance is common to this drug in south Asia, Pakistan, Kenya, and Nigeria. Treated children may continue to shed the bacteria in their stools and thus represent a risk of infection to others. Followup stool cultures upon return home are advised.

Families anticipating travel in south Asia and tropical Africa should consider vaccination against typhoid prior to departure. An oral vaccine is available with four doses over a 7 day period. Alternately there is an injectable vaccine that requires only one dose. Both vaccines require revaccination to maintain efficacy, and neither is 100% protective.

Abdominal pain

Entire textbooks have been devoted to the subject of abdominal pain in children. Although a comprehensive review of this subject would be beyond the scope of this book, some general guidelines are appropriate. Like most symptoms in children, "belly ache" must be considered in the physical and psychological context in which it occurs. The occasional complaint of non-specific abdominal discomfort IN THE ABSENCE OF OTHER SYMPTOMS is common and usually benign in children. Abdominal discomfort may precede the onset of gastroenteritis, or be associated with heartburn or acid indigestion in children with reflux. It may also be associated with the movement of large hard stool through the colon in children who are constipated. In each case, treatment of the offending condition will resolve the discomfort. Recurring complaints of non-specific mild abdominal discomfort in kids less than 10 years of age who do not have other symptoms are sufficiently common that you may observe the child without other interventions.

Vague non-increasing abdominal discomfort, with normal appetite, associated with loose stool, mucous, or traces of blood in the stool, but not with other signs of illness (lethargy, prostration, fever, etc) most likely represents infectious colitis. A stool sample should identify the offending agent and guide treatment.

On the other hand, INCREASING PERSISTENT abdominal pain may be associated with an emerging condition such as appendicitis. If abdominal pain is associated with loss of appetite, fever, or decreased stooling in a child free of chronic constipation, concern is warranted. On examination, if the abdomen is soft and gentle probing with your hand is not met with resistance or an increase in pain, this is reassuring. If the abdomen is tense, with tenderness to gentle pressure with your hand - particularly if that pressure is met with facial grimacing and increased tension, an intra-abdominal emergency may be developing. Likewise, if the sudden release of pressure by your hand causes an outcry and increase in pain, these signs indicate inflammation of the lining of the abdomen (peritonitis) - a very worrisome sign. Medical attention should be sought immediately, even if that requires evacuation.

Jaundice

Yellowish discoloration of the skin, also noticeable in the whites of the eyes in international travelers is most likely due to hepatitis (inflammation of the liver). The most likely cause is the hepatitis A virus, which is transmitted by contaminated food or water. Acute hepatitis A in children usually provokes no symptoms, goes unrecognized, and resolves completely. A small minority of children will develop clinical hepatitis with some degree of jaundice, mild lethargy, and decreased appetite. Infected children may transmit the disease to others for two weeks PRIOR to the development of jaundice and for one week afterward.

There is no chronic or carrier state. Immunization for hepatitis A virus is recommended in all children beyond 6 months of age with a booster dose 6-12 months thereafter. The vaccine is extremely effective. As a result, this infection which used to be common in children now occurs mostly in unvaccinated adults, who are more likely to develop jaundice. Unvaccinated adults may benefit from receiving a dose of immunoglobulin to prevent illness if exposed to a jaundiced child. Other causes of jaundice in children are vanishingly rare!

Diabetes

Type I diabetes develops predominately in childhood. Unless one or both parents have type I diabetes, the likelihood of a child developing this condition during travel is extremely small. Children develop diabetes over a period of weeks, during which time they exhibit increased urination, increased drinking of water, and weight loss despite adequate diet and appetite. 1/3 of such children will develop ketoacidosis, appear ill with lethargy and have the strong smell of acetone on their breath. Type I diabetics require insulin injections, and insulin must be continuously refrigerated, such children should not travel off the grid!

Pharyngitis (Sore Throat)

Most sore throats in children are associated with nasal congestion, but not with substantial fever and are due to virus infections. These illnesses will resolve spontaneously in 5-7 days and do not require specific treatment. Pharyngitis without cold symptoms, particularly with substantial fever and tender swollen lymph nodes below the corner of the jaw is more likely to be due to strep throat. Untreated strep throat may be complicated by acute rheumatic fever or kidney injury. For this reason, in the absence of a throat culture, you should ALWAYS treat severe sore throat with fever and swollen nodes with 10 days of Amoxicillin or Penicillin. Treatment hastens the resolution of symptoms and prevents the aforementioned complications. If the pharyngitis fails to respond to treatment, it may be due to Epstein Barr Virus infection, the cause of mononucleosis. Further antibiotic treatment is not beneficial in these cases, which will resolve spontaneously.

Otitis (Ear Pain)

Two types of ear pain occur in children: acute otitis externa and acute otitis media.

Otitis externa (swimmers ear) involves inflammation of the ear canal between the eardrum and external ear. It is not associated with fever or other signs of an upper respiratory viral infection. The diagnosis can be confirmed by pressing the soft tissue just in front of the ear canal while "wiggling" the ear. This will elecit pain in otitis externa. This condition is treated with antibiotic drops, preferably containing a steroid to reduce local inflammation (ie Ciprodex). Swimmers' ears can be avoided by rinsing both ear canals after swimming or showering with a 50:50 mixture of rubbing alcohol and white vinegar. This can be stored in a dropper or squirt bottle and does not require refrigeration.

Otitis Media usually occurs as a bacterial complication of a viral upper respiratory infection (cold) and is associated with the onset of fever and ear pain not worsened by the movement of the external ear. If the child has not had recurrent ear infections, Amoxicillin is given twice daily for 10 days. If the child has had previous ear infections a broader spectrum antibiotic such as Cefpodoxime or Amoxicillin clavulanate should be used. In some cases the eardrum may rupture, causing a yellowish or greenish discharge from the ear canal. This should resolve with effective treatment of the otitis media. If it does not resolve, irrigate the ear canal twice daily with hydrogen peroxide and treat it as otitis external with antibiotic ear drops.

Nosebleeds

The overwhelming majority of nosebleeds in children involve the anterior portion of the nasal septum and are caused by "digital manipulation", a fancy term for nose picking. Treatment of acute bleeding is simple, but the details are important. Hold the child's nose firmly between the thumb and forefinger, with the sides of the nostrils pressing against the nasal septum. This will compress the septum and stop further bleeding. You must hold this position for a minimum of five minutes to allow the irritated vessels to clot. Upon release discourage nose blowing, giving time for the area to heal. Failure of this treatment is rare and may indicate a posterior site of bleeding which must be treated by a physician. Recurrent nosebleeds are common and may be reduced by the use of an oral antihistamine for allergic rhinitis or simple saline nasal spray (OTC) applied four times daily for dry noses. If these are not effective the septal blood vessels will need to be cauterized by a physician.

<u>Cough</u>

Cough is a reflex, not an illness, and most often represents the body's response to inflammation in the nose and throat from a viral URI. Since it is an important aspect of the immune response, it should not be suppressed! Persistent or severe cough may be associated with fever, chest pain, wheezing, shortness of breath, etc. In such cases, it is the CAUSE of the cough that is important. Cough can generally be divided into upper and lower respiratory causes. Upper respiratory coughs are most often due to colds, although the presence of thick green or yellow nasal discharge FOR OVER TWO WEEKS, may indicate sinusitis. Colds begin with nasal congestion, followed after 2-3 days with a clear watery nasal discharge. After 3-5 days the discharge may become thick and yellow. Unless this change is associated with a change in the clinical status of the child (ie onset of ear pain or fever), the nature of the discharge only indicates that the immune system has mobilized white blood cells to combat the virus. The change from clear to green does NOT indicate a secondary bacterial infection, nor call for an antibiotic. Colds normally clear spontaneously within 7-10 days, so only if the thick discharge lasts for over two weeks do we consider sinusitis likely. Sinusitis is treated with 10-14 days of the same antibiotics used for acute otitis media (see above).

Laryngotracheal Bronchitis (Croup)

Viral Croup commonly affects children between 6 months and three years of age and involves inflammation of the airway below the vocal cords, producing hoarseness, and a barking cough (seal-like), associated with inspiratory "stridor". Stridor is produced by narrowing of the airway below the vocal cords, yet above the chest. It occurs when breathing in and is a coarse honking sound. Viral croup can produce significant respiratory distress and should be treated as soon as possible with a single dose of dexamethasone .6mg/kg. This will shorten the duration of the illness and relieve airway obstruction. If Dexamethasone is unavailable, a 5-day course of prednisone may be substituted.

In unimmunized children, a croupy cough associated with fever may represent Acute Epiglottitis. This illness is caused by an infection in the same area as croup, but with a bacteria (Haemophilus influenza type B). Epiglottitis is a very serious disease! Prior to the availability of an effective vaccine, this organism caused not only epiglottits, but cases of pneumonia, septic arthritis, and meningitis. The introduction of the vaccine reduced the incidence of H. influenza diseases by 99%, yet the ORGANISM still exists in the community. Treatment "off the grid" requires a dose of dexamethasone as in viral croup, as well as an antibiotic effective against H. Influenza (ie Azithromycin, Augmentin, or Cefixime). Even with rapid treatment, a fatality rate of over 10% can be expected - hence the absolute importance of vaccination!

Pneumonia

The overwhelming percentage of Lung infections in children are due to viruses and resolve spon-taneously. Cough may be worrisome, but these children do not appear substantially ill. The pres-ence of wheezing also suggests a viral process.

A child with a bacterial lung infection presents differently. These children appear terribly ill! They are lethargic with high fever and usually have pain in breathing, due to Inflammation of the lining of the chest wall. Breathing is shallow, rapid, and labored. Prior to antibiotics, bacterial pneumonia was almost always fatal. Now, these children are routinely treated as outpatients. Since you will not have an x-ray to confirm the diagnosis, you will have to trust the clinical signs. Within 24 hours of the initiation of appropriate antibiotic treatment (generally amoxicillin), the fever will subside and the child will no longer appear toxic. Treatment should continue for 7-10 days. With pneumonia, the breathing spaces of the lungs fill with pus. This is mobilized by the lining of the airways, brought up to the bronchi, and then expelled by coughing. Despite effective antibiotic treatment, the cough of pneumonia may persist, growing less only over weeks.

Wheezing and Asthma

Wheezes are high-pitched whistling sounds that emanate from the lungs and are heard most prominently on expiration (breathing out). Wheezing is the clinical hallmark of asthma, which is characterized by recurring episodes of cough, rapid breathing, and wheezing. The episodes are most often stimulated by viral URIs in childhood, although allergy becomes a more frequent precipitant in teens and adults.

The tendency to wheeze has a strong genetic component. Thus, cases of asthma tend to cluster in families. Any child with a history of wheezing in the past should not travel "off the grid" without an adequate supply of medications! During the initial 24-36 hours of an asthma episode, the predominant mechanism of airway obstruction is the contraction of the smooth muscles that surround the small airways of the lungs. Within 48 hours the dominant mechanism of airway obstruction becomes inflammation. This is important since the medications used to treat the two stages are different. During the initial stage, Albuterol, which is supplied as a nebulized mist directly into the airways will reverse the bronchial muscle spasm. It must be used early and vigorously to be effective. Albuterol is available in a metered dose inhaler (puffer), but this must be combined with a "spacer" if the medication is to reach the small airways. Spraying the medicine directly into the mouth is not effective, as most is deposited on the back of the throat and is swallowed. In the absence of a medical spacer, a homemade substitute can be fashioned by cutting the bottom out of a small plastic soft drink bottle. The cap end is held in the mouth of the patient while the metered dose inhaler is positioned at the large opening. The child holds his nose and takes a deep breath as the inhaler is fired. The dose for a child who is actively wheezing will be 3-5 puffs. This dose may be repeated every 15 minutes if the child is breathing rapidly or in distress. Thereafter dosage intervals should be increased, first to every 30 minutes, then hourly, then every 2-4 hours if the child has responded well. Albuterol lasts a maximum of 4 hours, and doses should be continued until all wheezing and cough have cleared. It is virtually impossible to "overdose" a child with albuterol. I have treated asthmatic children in distress with CONTINU-OUS inhaled albuterol for 24 hours, who would have otherwise required mechanical ventilation. The only side effect was a modest increase in heart rate. The child who continues to wheeze after 48 hours, will not respond adequately to albuterol, as the mechanism of airway obstruction has changed to swelling of the airway lining and increased secretion of mucous.

A systemic corticosteroid such as prednisone should be given to block inflammation. In most patients, this can be limited to five days, divided twice daily. Prednisone can be life-saving, and if limited to such short infrequent treatments, is free of side effects in children. If your child has had wheezing in the past, you should definitely carry both albuterol and prednisone on your travels.

Systemic Allergic Reactions

Anaphylaxis, a life-threatening allergic reaction (ie. Generally to foods such as peanuts or bee stings) occurs almost entirely in children who have a past history of previous reactions characterized by wheezing, difficulty breathing, and prostration. The parents of children with a history of systemic allergic reactions should already have an Epipen on hand and should travel with a supply of oral prednisone and an antihistamine (diphenhydramine or hydroxyzine). Hives, a raised itching rash that may move from one area to another and resolves over days, are treated with an antihistamine. Children with a history of hives are not at increased risk of more serious reactions, such as anaphylaxis.

<u>Insect Bites</u>

Mosquitos and other biting insects have evolved unique mechanisms for effectively feasting on our blood! Their mouthparts contain a sharp lance-like structure to puncture the skin and a thin tube to insert into the resulting wound. As our blood clots too rapidly for effective feeding, they have evolved an "anti-coagulant" (blood thinner) in their saliva, which is forcibly injected into the wound before taking their blood meal. It is our allergic response to the proteins in their saliva which causes the itching after mosquito bites. The organisms which cause malaria, zika, and west Nile fever all have life cycles within the mosquito which culminate in concentration within the mosquito's saliva. During feeding the mosquito transmits these pathogens to us via their saliva.

Allergic reactions to insect bites involve immune compounds within the skin that develop after exposure. Thus, when first bitten, no reaction occurs. Local reactions, particularly in young children, may be up to 5 inches in diameter, associated with severe swelling and itching, and require 3-7 days to resolve. Although dramatic, these reactions are not dangerous and can be treated with an oral antihistamine. Attention to the history of preceding insect bites and the absence of tenderness and warmth should avoid confusion with infection in the skin. Prolonged frequent exposure to the same species of insect bites may result in desensitization, wherein individuals no longer respond with an allergic reaction.

Avoidance of mosquitos, gnats, ticks, fleas, and biting flies involves wearing long-sleeved shirts and pants, gathered at the wrist and ankle, as well as head nets and sleeping under mosquito netting. Garments and mosquito nets pre-treated with insect repellants (ie. Insect Shield), as well as repellant that can be applied to garments (ie. Permethrin), are also available. Protective garments are moderately effective but may be uncomfortable in hot climates.

The addition of an insect repellant is advisable in areas where insect-borne diseases are prevalent. The gold standard of insect repellants is DEET, which is effective against mosquitos, biting flies, chiggers, fleas, and ticks and has been used safely for over 75 years. Although available in concentrations of 10-75 %, products with more than 30% DEET are not more effective. 10% of products provide protection for about 2 hours. Protection may be extended to 5 hours by 24% concentrations. 10-35% DEET has been shown to be safe in children > 2 months of age if used appropriately. Read labels carefully and follow the instructions. Use the lowest concentration for the expected exposure and bath thereafter. Worldwide fewer than 20 reports of toxicity from DEET have been reported in children. All such cases were associated with children ingesting DEET or with excessive prolonged application of highly concentrated products. Products containing both DEET and sunscreen should be avoided as reapplication for sun protection may result in excessive dosing with DEET.

Bed bugs live in the crevices of mattresses and their associated bedclothes, and are common in economically depressed areas. They come out at night to feed on unsuspecting guests, take their blood meal, and then disappear. Bites appear as small itchy bumps, which resolve if not scratched. Bed bugs do not transmit disease to humans but are a nuisance. DEET is not effective for bed bugs.

Skin Infections:

Our skin represents the largest "organ" in the body. Specialized sweat glands keep us cool, while the stratified epithelial surface presents a border with the outside world, protecting us from dehydration, injury, and invasion by bacteria. When the horny outer layers of the skin are interrupted by cuts, abrasions, or insect bites, bacteria can gain entrance into the subcutaneous tissues. Specialized enzymes secreted by the invaders dissolve the linkage between cells, allowing bacteria to spread through subcutaneous spaces, muscle, and bone and enter the bloodstream. The spectrum of skin Infections extends from superficial Impetigo to cellulitis, deep space abscesses, and the dreaded "flesh-eating" infections.

Impetigo

Bacterial infection of the skin is a common problem in hot humid climates. Impetigo represents a mixed infection with Strep and Staph organisms and presents as weeping tender lesions, which subsequently crust. The most common source of bacteria is the anterior nose. We all rub and pick at our noses from time to time, transporting bacteria to our fingernails in the process. When we scratch mosquito and other insect bites, we literally plow the bacteria into the skin. Within the skin, our local immune system releases chemical mediators that dilate capillaries (causing redness and heat) and summon white blood cells to the area to engulf the bacteria. If the local immune response is overwhelmed, cells begin to break down producing a weeping lesion full of rapidly reproducing bacteria - impetigo. Picking at infected skin lesions can rapidly spread the infection to new sites. If less than four infected lesions are present, they may be washed with soap and water, dressed with a topical antibiotic cream, and covered with a bandaid or dressing. This prevents the child from picking at the lesions and spreading the infection. The best topical antibiotic cream is Mupirocin (Bactroban). Children's fingernails should be trimmed very short!

If the infection continues to spread deeper invasion may occur and an oral antibiotic will be needed. The drug of choice is Clindamycin, which covers resistant Staph as well as Strep. Local treatment should continue until all lesions are crusted and dry.

Cellulitis

Once the skin barrier is disrupted and localized infection is established, rapidly reproducing Strep bacteria spread into the subcutaneous space. There the bacterial enzymes break cellular bonds, allowing the infection to spread horizontally, and to deeper layers. This presents as an expanding area of redness that is raised, tender and warm to the touch, a war zone between the army of bacteria and the body's immune response - in which the bacteria are clearly winning! The surface skin is usually dry and free of lesions. If the process is not treated promptly with antibiotics covering Strep and Staph, invasion of deeper structures may occur, leading to infection of muscle and bone or invasion of the bloodstream. Once again, Clindamycin is an excellent drug for cellulitis.

Abscess

If the immune response halts the progress of the infection within the sub-cutaneous tissue, migration of white blood cells and inflammatory "cytokines" into the mass circumscribing its spread. The resulting mass of bacteria, white blood cells, and cellular breakdown products becomes "walled off" from the surrounding tissue, producing an abscess. This presents as a tender inflamed nodule or mass within the subcutaneous space, which may be firm or soft. The abscess represents the victorious outcome of the local immune response and will "burrow" slowly to the surface. When the abscess "points" at the surface, the thinnest portion should be incised with a scalpel or other clean sharp instrument, and the pus allowed to drain. Sterility is not critical, as the area is already grossly infected and the immune response is activated. Complete drainage of the abscess heralds the end of the process, as it will continue to heal without antibiotic treatment.

Fungal Skin Infections

Fungal skin infections are generally superficial, occurring in the moist warm areas between adjacent skin surfaces, such as between toes, in the groin or diaper area, and between the chin and chest of young children. Areas between adjacent skin surfaces may become macerated (wet).

The most common organisms are yeast such as Candida in the diaper area and neck of infants. Candida rashes respond well to Nystatin cream, applied 2-3 times daily. Macerated lesions that have become foul smelling may be secondarily infected with skin bacteria and require concomitant topical anti-fungal and oral antibiotic treatment. On areas of dry skin, the classic "ringworm" lesion may occur. This shows an advancing inflamed area with central clearing. Ringworm is most commonly due to dermatophyte infection in older children.

Dermatophyte infections may be treated topically with a variety of Azole medications, such as Miconazole, Ketoconazole, Clotrimazole, and others for up to 4 weeks. Infections occurring in hair-bearing areas (scalp and groin) require oral treatment with terbinafine, fluconazole, or griseofulvin. Fungi infections require relatively prolonged treatment, often for 3-4 weeks to obtain complete resolution.

Lacerations

Superficial cuts through the skin can be repaired with adhesive tape. While still bleeding, irrigate the wound with clean water to remove any foreign material. The most effective way to halt bleeding is by the application of pressure directly to the cut with a clean cloth or sterile pad. Unless a blood vessel has been severed, bleeding should stop within five minutes. Do not remove the pad until five minutes have elapsed to avoid pulling off any clotted blood and renewing bleeding. Cut a number of tape strips approximately 2 inches long. When bleeding has stopped, carefully clean the surface with soap and water, and allow it to air dry. When dry, begin adjacent to one end of the cut, placing 1 inch of tape on the far side of the cut, at 90 degrees, and snug it to the skin. Pull gently on the tape, approximating the edges of the cut, and press the tape down on the near side. Place a similar tape near the opposite end of the cut. Working from alternate ends, continue adding tape until the wound is completely closed, leaving a small gap between each successive tape. Cover the tape and wound loosely with a clean gauze pad and tape strips.

Remove the pad daily to inspect the wound. A small amount of puffiness or redness at the wound margins is acceptable. Should the wound experience increasing redness, swelling, and tenderness, it has become infected. If the swelling is maximal at one point, carefully remove the tape over that section and allow it to drain. Giving a 5-7 day course of Amoxicillin/clavulanate or clindamycin may speed resolution, but need not be given unless wound infection occurs.

Keep the wound clean and dry, leave tape strips in place for 10-14 days, at which time they may be carefully removed.

Puncture Wounds

Puncture wounds and crush injuries represent a high risk of infection with Clostridium tetani, the causative agent of tetanus (lockjaw). If children have received their routine vaccinations, followed by a tetanus booster every 10 years, the risk of tetanus is negligible. Such wounds should be copiously irrigated with clean water prior to dressing. If the last tetanus booster was greater than 5 years prior to the injury a booster should be obtained. Children who have not been vaccinated should receive tetanus immune globulin as well as tetanus vaccination from a local clinic or hospital if they sustain a puncture wound or crush injury. Once tetanus presents clinically it is not treatable and frequently fatal.

If a child sustains a DEEP puncture wound THROUGH A SPORT OR TENNIS SHOE, there is a substantial risk of infection with pseudomonas, an organism that thrives in the insole of shoes. Observe the wound daily. If ANY redness or swelling occurs, give a 5-7 day course of Ciprofloxacin. Once established pseudomonas infections of the foot are very difficult to treat, requiring surgical drainage and IV antibiotics.

<u>Fish Hook Removal</u>

If a barbed fish hook is buried in the flesh, a simple maneuver makes removal quick and virtually painless but requires courage on the part of both patient and operator. Obtain a two-foot length of monofilament line or dental floss. Tie the line into a loop and slip this over the free end of the hook, adjusting its position such that the string lies against the curve of the hook, with the slack section beyond the hook (see illustration). Apply gentle pressure downward on the shank of the hook (the section between the eye and the curve) at an angle of 90 degrees. This disengages the barb from the flesh and creates a passage for its removal. Grasp the free end of the loop with the other hand, leaving a slack line between the hand and hook. Distract the patient briefly and pull sharply on the string. The hook will spring free. If the operators' effort is timid, the barb will catch, creating pain and the patient will be unlikely to tolerate a second attempt.

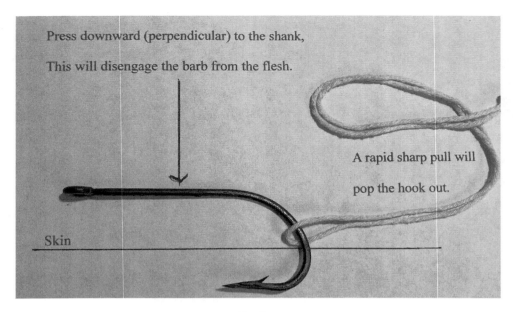
Caption

Burns

A traumatic injury may result from contact with a hot object, or liquid, chemicals, friction, radiation, or an electrical discharge. The resulting injury to the skin and subcutaneous tissues have classically been described as first, second, third, or fourth-degree burns.

Superficial first-degree burns, such as mild sunburns damage only the outer layers of the skin. They appear red, dry, and blanch to digital pressure. They are painful and tender to touch. They heal within 3-6 days without treatment, although an aloe or Lidocaine-containing cream may provide pain relief.

Superficial second-degree burns involve the epidermis and upper dermis, producing blisters, which yield a red weeping base if unroofed. These burns also blanch with pressure, are painful to contact, and heal within 7-21 days if no infection occurs.

Deep second-degree burns involve injury to the entire epidermis and dermis. They blister and produce wet weeping bases, but do not blanch with pressure. Islands of reproducing cells exist around sweat glands and hair follicles, from which healing occurs. Healing may take over 21 days and will result in significant scarring.

Third-degree burns involve the entire epidermis and dermis, with the complete destruction of skin structures. These wounds are NOT sensitive to touch and heal by scar formation from the periphery. Third-degree burns are generally treated by surgical skin grafting.

Fourth-degree burns involve the destruction of the skin, and subcutaneous fat, extending into the underlying fascia and muscle. These injuries require surgical treatment.

Treatment of minor burns

NEVER put ice on a burn, as it will extend the injury by reducing blood flow. Minor burns can be cooled with clean tap water. Once brought to room temperature further cooling is not beneficial. If blisters appear they should be left unbroken if possible, as they provide a sterile dressing for the underlying tissue. Once broken, the wet burn surface is subject to contamination and should be gently washed with soap and water. Any blister fragments or necrotic tissue should be removed and a dressing with silver sulfadiazine cream, covered by a non-adhesive gauze applied. This dressing is removed daily to inspect the wound. Clean partial thickness burns can be covered with xeroform gauze, which binds to the burn surface, reducing the frequency and discomfort of dressing changes. Large or full-thickness burns should be cleaned with soap and water, dressed with a bulky gauze dressing, and brought to medical attention as soon as possible. If medical evaluation and treatment must be delayed, the wound should be covered with silver sulfadiazine cream, adaptic or xeroform gauze, and a bulky dressing. This dressing should be changed and the wound cleansed daily. Large area burns represent a risk of dehydration due to the drainage exhibit. All significant burns should be brought to medical attention as soon as possible.

Head Injuries

Closed head injuries can occur in falls and when the head is struck by a moving object. Although most falls less than 10 ft. do not cause brain injury, all children who sustain a head injury should be observed closely. A brief seizure occurring at the time of the injury, may not be clinically significant if the child has no prolonged unconsciousness. On the other hand, seizures, or persistent vomiting that occur in the post-injury period as well as any PROGRESSIVE change in the level of consciousness or behavior (irritability or lethargy) may indicate serious injury. Further evaluation requires CT scans not available "off the grid" as well as access to neurosurgical treatment. Any child who has sustained a head injury and shows deterioration should be evacuated.

Residual symptoms after an acute head injury may indicate a concussion. These include headache, dizziness, difficulty concentrating, confusion, nausea, drowsiness, and sensitivity to noise and light. Treatment involves rest in a quiet non-stimulating environment. If symptoms progress, or do not resolve within 2-3 weeks, evacuation should be considered.

Seizures

Seizures represent a spontaneous disorganized discharge in the brain which most commonly produces an alteration in consciousness associated with rhythmic, non-purposeful movements such as shaking or jerking. The vast majority of seizures are not in themselves dangerous but are frightening to bystanders. Obviously, a seizure that occurs while a child is in a vulnerable situation, such as swimming, can be lethal. Children with poorly controlled seizure disorders should not travel off the grid. On the other hand, a child whose seizure disorder is well controlled on medication should be at minimally increased risk, so long as an adequate supply of medication is available. Although it is extremely unlikely that a child would develop a seizure disorder during travel that had not previously expressed itself, there are exceptions that deserve consideration.

Febrile Seizures

2-4% of children less than 5 years of age may experience a brief seizure associated with fever. The peak incidence occurs between 12 and 18 months of age. The underlying illness may be a simple viral infection. Such seizures are generally brief, lasting less than 5 minutes, but may on occasion last up to 15 minutes. The child is unconscious and is not aware of the episode. Febrile seizures are felt to be due to immaturity of the developing nervous system, are not dangerous, and do not portend future epilepsy. If a young child with a fever develops seizure activity, do not attempt to restrain their movements or put anything in the mouth. After the seizure has passed, attend to the cause. The child may appear confused or drowsy, but this should clear rapidly. What other symptoms is the child having? You may want to treat the fever with Acetaminophen (Tylenol) and after 20-30 minutes, with cool compresses or a bath. Children who have a substantial fever and are treated with cooling baths BEFORE Tylenol has had time to be effective may experience "shaking chills" or shivering which parents may mistakenly confuse with a seizure.

Seizures with CNS Infection

Any child who has a seizure with fever and a decreased or altered level of consciousness may be developing meningitis or encephalitis. Such children usually will have experienced lethargy or agitation associated with fever BEFORE the seizure, but the seizure activity may be the first sign of brain infection. Any child with a progressive alteration in consciousness associated with fever must be brought to medical attention as soon as possible. Infection of the covering of the brain (meningoencephalitis) may be due to viral or bacterial infection. Viral encephalitis occurs worldwide, is usually mild and not dangerous, and does not respond to antibiotic treatment.

Bacterial meningitis may be rapidly fatal if not treated! If you are unable to obtain evacuation in a timely manner, I would recommend initiating antibiotic therapy, although this may make subsequent diagnosis more difficult. The most frequent causes of bacterial meningitis in children are all treated with IV antibiotics, which will not be available to you. The combination of high doses (100 mg/kg every 12 hours) of Amoxicillin and Chloramphenicol (not available in the U.S.) will cover the most likely pathogens, while you continue to pursue evacuation!

Seizures associated with trauma

Rarely a brief seizure may occur at the time of a blow to the head. If this lasts less than 5 minutes and the child returns to a normal level of consciousness thereafter, the child should be observed closely and attention should be directed to other signs of injury. If there is prolonged or progressive lethargy, or if the seizure occurs minutes to hours after the trauma, the risk of serious traumatic brain injury warrants immediate medical evaluation or evacuation.

Dislocations Common dislocations in children involve the shoulder and elbow.

Nursemaids Elbow

Anterior dislocation of the elbow (nursemaids elbow) occurs in children less than five years of age when an adult pulls on the child's wrist with the arm fully extended. It may also occur when the child's wrist is held and the child drops, such as during a temper tantrum.

Pain is immediate and the child refuses to move the arm, holding it against the body with the palm turned partially downward. There should be no swelling, tenderness, or discoloration along the bones of the lower arm or wrist. Attempts to turn the wrist palm upward produce immediate pain and resistance.

The forearm consists of two parallel bones, the radius, and ulna. With the palm facing upward, the Ulna extends from the medial aspect of the wrist to the point of the elbow. The Radius extends from the lateral side of the wrist (palm up) to the lateral side of the elbow. In nursemaids' elbow, the head of the radius is displaced from the elbow joint. Reduction is uncomfortable but simple enough to be carried out by an adult. Facing the child, who is seated and gently restrained in a parent's lap, the operator sits facing the child.

Holding the elbow gently with the opposite hand, place the thumb over the head of the radius, applying gentle pressure. While applying traction to the wrist (pulling on the arm), simultaneously turn the child's palm upward and flex the elbow. A "click" will be felt beneath the operator's thumb as the head of the radius slips back into position. Within 5-10 minutes the child will use their arm normally (See illustration below)

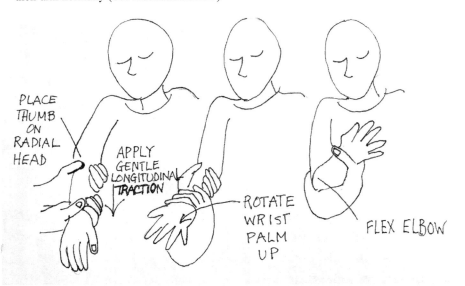

Treatment of anterior dislocation of radial head in children

Shoulder Dislocation:

Anterior shoulder dislocation occurs in children over 10 years of age or adults, secondary to a blow to the back of the upper arm or a fall on the extended arm. The shoulder loses its rounded contour as the head of the upper arm bone (humerus) is displaced anteriorly from the shoulder socket. Pain may be intense and the patient will resist movement of the affected shoulder. This muscle spasm makes reduction (return of the head of the humerus into the shoulder socket) more difficult. In children, the risk of an associated fracture or vascular compromise in the joint is very low, and attempted reduction by a parent "off the grid" is reasonable.

Complications are possible, but quite rare. If pain and the resulting spasm cause the reduction to fail, and medical facilities are not available, it is reasonable to give a single dose of a sedative to relieve anxiety and spasm prior to repeated attempts at reduction. Leaving the shoulder dislocated is not acceptable due to the pain and risk of permanent injury to the joint.

All sedatives and narcotic pain relievers carry a small risk of depression of the respiratory drive. Given as a single agent in the appropriate dosage, Midazolam (Versed) has minimal risk. It is not a pain reliever but is moderately sedating and relieves anxiety. It also produces retrograde amnesia of the event. The patient will be able to cooperate in the reduction and may complain of pain, but will not remember the incident.

Midazolam should be given ONLY ONCE, by mouth or by instillation into the nose. Onset occurs within 20 minutes and the duration of effect does not exceed one hour. Respiratory rate

should be observed, giving cues to breathe if the rate falls below 20/min. Although sedative/hypnotic or narcotic agents would generally be used ONLY under the controlled conditions of ambulatory surgery, emergency room, or physician's office, exceptional situations "off the grid" warrant their careful use. Obviously, the medication would have to be purchased in advance in order to be available when you are far from medical help. You will also have to assume the risk associated with its use! It could also be of use in treating a significant laceration or burn injury.

Numerous mechanisms for reduction are described. My preference is as follows: the teen lies on his back with the elbow at his side, flexed to 90 degrees. While the elbow is held snugly against the body by the operator's hand, the operator holds the teen's wrist with his other hand and very slowly and gently allows the lower arm to rotate away from the body. Whenever muscle spasms or pain occur the movement is stopped and the arm allowed to relax.

Gradually, over 5-10 minutes, the arm rotates sufficiently (usually 70-110 degrees) to allow the head of the humorous to reduce. This may be associated with a "clunk", felt by the operator. Reduction is confirmed by the patient being able to place his hand on the opposite shoulder. The arm should be placed in a sling and kept immobilized for 2-3 weeks.

Fractures

Our bones represent dynamic living tissue, capable of significant spontaneous healing after insult. The stiff mineral component of bones is covered by a membrane (periosteum) with a rich supply of blood vessels. Injury is followed by three stages of healing: inflammatory, reparative, and remodeling. When a bone breaks, the periosteum is torn, leading to a blood clot surrounding the fracture site. Cells from the clot, and from new vessels that grow into the fracture site, develop into a fibrous callus, which is initially cartilaginous. During the reparative stage, osteocytes begin to lay down new bone in the callus, leading to a boney union of the fracture.

At this point, the fracture site is no longer tender and the extremity can be used without significant pain. In the remodeling stage, a balance between bone deposition and reabsorption reshapes the callus to yield a fully repaired bone. Since children remodel their entire skeleton each year, remodeling proceeds rapidly in the young.

Most fractures are "closed" in which there is no penetration of the skin by the bone fragments. There will be swelling and tenderness at the fracture site, as well as pain if the distal fragment is moved. In simple closed fractures the two segments of bone remain aligned, with minimal angulation or overlap. The initial management of a simple closed fracture entails stabilization of the fracture site, accomplished at home by casting. Off the grid, it will require splinting with strips of wood or plastic. The extremity should first be padded with a cloth to avoid pressure points and the splints over-wrapped with elastic bandages or strips of cloth. The extremity must be immobi lized throughout the reparative stage, as any movement of the fracture segments will retard healing.

Broken fingers can be splinted with a tongue depressor or Popsicle stick extending onto the back of the hand and by taping them to the adjacent finger. A fractured toe may simply be taped to an adjacent uninjured toe. Even simple closed fractures should be brought to the attention of a physician as soon as possible, but their initial stabilization and treatment may be managed "off the grid".

In open fractures, a bone fragment penetrates the skin. This requires much more movement of the fracture segments and normally occurs only with extreme trauma. Even if the bone were successfully reduced, the wound has a high risk of infection and such injuries warrant immediate evacuation.

Urinary Tract Infections

Due to their anatomy, bladder infections (cystitis) occur almost entirely in girls. With the exception of cases of recurrent or chronic infection, the causative bacteria, E. Coli, derive from the GI tract. Infection of the bladder causes irritation of the bladder wall and urethra, leading to the cardinal symptoms of UTI: urgency, frequency, and painful voiding.

The bladder is composed of muscle fibers. When it is inflamed it contracts forcefully long before it is full. This leads to an increase in the frequency of voiding. associated with feelings of urgency. Inflammation of the urethra causes stinging pain during voiding. Infection limited to the bladder does not cause fever, and symptoms beyond the bladder are usually absent.

Acute kidney infection - which is far less common, causes fever, systemic illness, and flank tenderness, as well as the lower urinary symptoms of bladder infection. Unlike simple bladder infection, kidney infection carries the risk of scarring and loss of kidney function if not treated promptly.

Recommended treatment for simple cystitis in the past has relied on amoxicillin and Bactrim, however, increased frequency of resistant organisms has prompted a change to newer antibiotics. At the time of writing, the choice of experts is cefuroxime or cefprozil, for cystitis, although cefdinir or cefixime are also good choices. Cefixime (Suprax) has the advantage of being available as chewable tablets and is indicated for both cystitis and acute kidney infection. Whichever drug is chosen, treatment should be continued for 7-14 days for kidney infection. Infection limited to the bladder may be stopped after 5 days.The symptoms of cystitis can be quickly relieved by administration of phenazopyridine (Pyridium) which is available over the counter in the U.S. This medication should be used for no longer than 2 days (along with antibiotic treatment) to avoid masking symptoms of treatment failure. Follow-up urinalysis or culture are not necessary if symptoms resolve promptly. Any child with continued symptoms should consult a local medical facility.

VulvoVaginitis

_The vulva and vaginal tract of prepubertal girls are lined with epithelium as delicate as that lining your eyes. Under the influence of pubertal hormones, this thickens and develops secretions that protect it from infection and inflammation. The absence of any structural barrier between the anus and vulva leaves the area open to contamination with fecal bacteria during wiping or from tight-fitting underwear. Vulvovaginitis produces burning during urination, which may be confused with a bladder infection. The former is NOT associated with urgency or frequency. In fact, young girls with vaginitis will try to prolong the intervals between voiding to avoid the associated discomfort. They can easily sleep through the night, whereas cystitis shows no respect for sleep! Finally, girls with vaginitis may have a yellowish discharge that often appears on their underwear, unlikely with cystitis. The primary treatment of vulvar inflammation in prepubertal girls is sitz baths, not antibiotics. Sitting for 15-20 minutes is a bath or basin of clean warm water, waving the water into the area of the vulva three to four times daily allows healing within 2-3 days in almost all cases. This also provides the child with a painless opportunity to void. Initially, the mom should gently inspect the area between the labia for the presence of bruising or foreign material. Never use soap on the genital area of prepubertal girls, avoid bubble baths and wear light cotton underwear. Review hygiene with the child, emphasizing careful front-to-back wiping after bowel movements. If symptoms do not resolve after 3-5 days of sitz baths, or if the discharge persists, a 7-day course of amoxicillin may be needed.

Labial adhesions represent a longer-term complication of even minimal vulvar irritation. This occurs when an epithelial bridge forms between the labia, which subsequently fuse. Unless complete fusion occurs, blocking the passage of urine, this is a minor problem, usually noted on inspection by a parent. It may be tempting to simply pull the labia apart - DON'T! The application of conjugated estrogen (Premarin) cream twice daily allows the epithelium to "mature" and the labia will separate painlessly.

Vaginitis in teens may be due to irritation from masturbation, soaps, or hygiene products, but more likely represents an infection. Sitz baths and a review of hygiene products may solve the problem. If not, consideration of the most likely infectious agents is in order. If the teen has a thick white odorless curd-like vaginal discharge with significant itching, candida infection is likely. Oral treatment with a single 150 mg dose of fluconazole is effective in over 90%. If itching is not present and the discharge is thin, malodorous, and grey in color, bacterial vaginosis is likely. This represents a complex alteration in the vaginal ecosystem which resolves spontaneously in over 30% of cases. Other causes of vaginal discharge in sexually active teens include STDs and will require consultation with a clinic capable of performing cultures.

Regional considerations

Illnesses follow distributions that reflect climate or insect vector distributions. Thus illnesses found in tropical areas of Central America, the Caribbean, Northern Australia, the SW Pacific, and South Asia do not occur in the temperate zones to their north and south. When planning your trip you should review the zones through which you will be traveling and the disease risks in those areas. Most risk can be minimized through insect avoidance, the use of protective clothing, wearing shoes, avoiding exposure to infected freshwater sources, exercising care with food and water, and prophylactic treatment for Malaria, where indicated.

Australia, New Zealand and the SW Pacific

These destinations can be divided into tropical and temperate climatic zones, with differing health concerns. Northern Australia, unlike the southern temperate zone, is tropical, sparsely populated, and has few hospitals. It shares these characteristics with the islands of the western pacific, a major destination for cruising sailors, where the population is sparse and widely separated. Medical facilities are generally located near population centers and tourist destinations. Temperate southern Australia and the entirety of New Zealand have sophisticated medical services and well-developed communications.

Temperate Australia and New Zealand

Health concerns in the temperate zone are similar to the continental U.S. Urban water supplies are safe to drink and food supplies are inspected. Ross River Fever and Barmah Forest Virus infections are transmitted by mosquitos, are most common during the summer (December - February), and prompt the use of insect repellant. These viruses cause fever, headache, muscle aches, rash, and fatigue. They are not treatable but generally resolve without sequelae.

Australian Tick Typhus occurs throughout the eastern coastal area and is transmitted by tick bites. (See section on Rickettsial diseases). Campers and hikers are most at risk, and the highest prevalence is during the dry season (June - November). The illness presents with fever, rash, headache, and muscle pain. Murine typhus also occurs in temperate Australia, and the north island of New Zealand, and is transmitted by flea bites. Scrub typhus is also present, which is transmitted by chigger bites. Leptospirosis occurs throughout rural eastern Australia and is most often associated with the dairy and beef industries. Thus these diseases may be acquired during "home stays", or recreational exposure to fresh water.

This may sound confusing and frightening, so let's simplify. All these infections have similarly non-specific symptoms. In the USA your doctor would sort them out using blood tests, that are not available to you off the grid. The infections fall into two categories: viral and rickettsial. Viral infections do not respond to treatment, but are generally less dangerous and will resolve with out medication. Rickettsia and the spirochetes of Leptospirosis respond to Doxycycline, generally showing rapid improvement. Off the grid, in an isolated area of temperate Australia, if you develop fever, headache, myalgia, and rash, take 7 days of Doxycycline! It's the same thing your doctor at home would recommend pending the results of blood tests! After 3-5 days, if the child's condition is not improving, urgent local consultation would be required. If persistently worse, evacuate to a medical center.

Marine Risks

Australian waters are home to the Box Jellyfish, which are most prevalent between October and May. Contact with the tentacles releases a neurotoxin, which can cause cardiac arrest within 5 minutes! Heed posted warnings, and stay out of the ocean if jellyfish are present. Snorkeling the reefs of eastern Australia is the stuff of legends, and should not be missed, but avoid handling marine creatures that you do not recognize. The spines of the beautiful Lionfish produce painful stings, while the bite of the Blue Ringed Octopus may be lethal.

Ciguatera (fish poisoning) occurs when the flesh of an affected fish is consumed. The toxin is concentrated in carnivorous fish, being most likely in larger fish that feed around coral reefs such as Barracuda, or large snapper. The toxin is tasteless and there is no reliable test for its presence. Symptoms include changes in mental status, weakness, hallucinations, a metallic taste in the mouth, and difficulty walking, as well as vomiting, diarrhea, and cramps, all occurring within three days of ingestion. Recovery is the general rule, but some symptoms may persist for weeks to months. Following local recommendations on which fish are safe to eat is reasonable.

<u>North Australia and SW Pacific Islands</u>

North and central Australia are hot, vast, and dry. Roads are often of poor quality and medical facilities are widely separated. Every year individuals die in the "outback" due to dehydration so plan accordingly. Many islands of the SW pacific are poorly developed, making access to medical support difficult. Travelers over land or by sea need to prepare and plan carefully to anticipate and support their medical needs.

Tropical North Australia and the SW pacific islands share many of the health risks of temperate Australia, including Typhus, Leptospirosis, and various mosquito-borne virus infections. Dengue fever virus occurs throughout the region as well as Chikungunya Virus infection. All these viruses are untreatable but may be avoided by the use of protective clothing and mosquito repellant. In the presence of fever, rash, headache, and myalgia it is reasonable to begin a course of Doxycycline and observation. If improvement does not follow, local medical consultation should be sought. Health risks limited to the region include Australian Bat lyssavirus infection, which is similar to rabies and occurs after direct contact with infected bats. Large fruit-eating bats are consumed by islanders. Do not handle bats! A post-exposure vaccine is available for those bitten or scratched.

Snails and slugs carry the rat lungworm, Angiostrongylus. Infection can be transmitted by eating unwashed leafy vegetables and fruits as well as by ingestion of the snail, This may lead to meningitis. No treatment is available, but the illness resolves. Avoidance is obviously the key. While working in American Samoa I saw over a hundred cases of this disease within one year, mostly in children. All survived intact, with only supportive care. Severe infection was limited to those who ate the snails.

Dog hookworm is common throughout the tropics and may be avoided by wearing shoes. The larval stage of the worm penetrates the skin to establish infection. Do not go barefoot, particularly in and around villages.

Tuberculosis occurs throughout the region but is most often transmitted during prolonged close contact, such as within families. Casual contact by travelers is considered low risk, but precautions should be taken by those planning extended stays in homes or villages.

Hepatitis A is endemic (always present), but travelers should be protected by their immunization. Jaundice, if present is usually mild.

Typhoid fever is common throughout the tropics, occurring when Salmonella species are ingested with contaminated food or water. After 1-3 weeks, patients develop prolonged fever, chills, abdominal pain, and rash. Diarrhea occurs in only about half of the cases. Diagnosis requires stool culture. Presumptive treatment is reasonable in children traveling in endemic areas with symptoms that are consistent and fever for more than 3 days. Because the organism has become resistant to other antibiotics, the drug of choice is now Azithromycin for 7 days. Typhoid vaccine may be recommended prior to travel through endemic areas. Discuss this with your doctor.

Malaria exists throughout the tropics, however, the risk is greatest in rural areas during periods of high rainfall. The most serious disease is caused by Falciparum malaria. This presents with high fever (>104 degrees F.) and delirium in the absence of other explanatory symptoms. Unlike the classic picture of malaria which presents as recurring indolent fever and night sweats, Falciparum malaria can rapidly lead to shock, brain swelling, organ failure, and death. Prevention is critical. Consult the Centers for Disease Controls recommendations for travelers for your planned itinerary, found at wwwnc.cdc.gov/travel/diseases/malaria. The frequency of drug resistance, organisms seen and recommended medications for prophylaxis vary between islands throughout the SW Pacific and must be followed. Because malaria can progress so rapidly, mosquito avoidance is strongly advised (see Insect Bites), but not sufficient in many areas. Pregnant women are at particularly high risk of life-threatening infection, stillbirth, and abortion and should delay travel to malarious areas until after delivery.

Preventive (prophylactic) medications for malaria in children include Atovaquone/proguanil (Malarone) and Mefloquine. Mefloquine has the advantage of being dosed once a week but has more frequent side effects. Doxycycline taken daily is effective but may cause sun sensitization. Falciparum malaria is resistant to chloroquine in many areas. If resistance is low in your travel area, Chloroquine may be used for prophylaxis.

Whichever medication is chosen, it should be started prior to entering the malarious area and continued for a period (depending on the medication used) after leaving it. Review your planned itinerary, check the current CDC list, and stock up on prophylactic medication before you embark. It may not be available in-country.

Uncomplicated malaria can be treated with Atovaquone/proguanil, or Doxycycline with Quinine (see appendix for doses). Presumptive treatment may be necessary if lab facilities are not available.

Melioidosis is caused by infection with soil bacteria. It is hyperendemic in North Australia, also occurring in NE Thailand. Most infections occur during the rainy monsoon season and remain asymptomatic. 95% of acute cases occur in adults, where the organism may cause pneumonia. Only 5% of acute infections occur in children, presenting as skin abscesses, which fail to heal with routine treatment. Since the organism can cause chronic or recurrent disease years after the initial infection, all patients are treated with a course of IV antibiotics, followed by 3-6 months of two oral antibiotics. The illness would be suspected in a child with an abscess that fails to resolve on treatment (see Skin infections), or which was followed by fever and systemic illness. Blood tests are available for travelers who suspect they may have contracted the illness. Cases in travelers are uncommon but have been documented.

South Asia

This area includes the Philippines, Borneo, Indonesia, New Guinea, Malaysia, Myanmar, Thailand, Laos, Cambodia, Viet Nam, India, and Pakistan. Because there is great variation, not only between countries but between rural and urban areas within each country, reliance on the CDC and WHO websites for international travelers is highly recommended. Consideration of the details of each area would be far beyond the scope of this book.

In general, urban centers within the region are far less likely to represent risks of tropical or infectious diseases. Malaria may be endemic in rural areas but non-existent in cities. Mosquitos, ticks, and fleas may not be present, and being run over by a rickshaw or motorbike may rank higher on your list of dangers. If one plans extended visits to villages or rural areas precautions for TB exposure, malaria, and other tropical and insect-borne diseases may be prudent. If travel is restricted to urban areas such precautions are generally unnecessary.

Resistance of Malaria to Mefloquine in south Asian countries prompts the use of Atovaquone/ proguanil or Doxycycline for prophylaxis. As in previously covered tropical areas Dengue, various mosquito-borne viral infections, typhoid fever, leptospirosis, and cholera are all endemic to the area, but the risk to travelers is much lower than to nationals. Mosquito avoidance is clearly warranted.

Diseases transmitted by freshwater include leptospirosis and schistosomiasis. Leptospirosis infection follows exposure to water contaminated with animal urine. This disease also occurs in the subtropical U.S., including the states of Florida and Hawaii. Risk factors include recreational swimming, canoeing, kayaking, and walking barefoot through the water. Outbreaks have occurred following triathlons in the U.S., Europe, and Asia. While most infections remain asymptomatic, acute illness may occur within 1-3 wks. after infection, and presents with fever, chills, muscle pain, and headache. Conjunctival redness or hemorrhage are common and help differentiate it from other non-specific febrile illnesses. After an initial 2-9 days of fever, the child may appear to improve, but the return of fever heralds the onset of the "immune" phase of the disease. During this phase meningitis, pneumonia and respiratory failure, kidney disease, extreme muscle tenderness, and neurologic findings may occur. Since diagnosis requires lab testing not available "off the grid", treatment should begin within two days of onset with Doxycycline or Azithromycin. This is felt to shorten the illness and reduce the risk of progression to severe disease.

Schistosomiasis is present in Vietnam, Cambodia, Laos, the southern islands of the Philippines, and the Yangtze River basin of China, and is transmitted through contact with fresh water. Infection can occur after a single contact, and outbreaks have been associated with tourism. The infectious larvae penetrate intact skin and migrate to the liver, where the adult worms may live in a perpetual cycle of egg laying for decades. Penetration of the skin by free-swimming larvae is followed by an itching rash, most commonly on the feet and lower legs (swimmer's itch). Travelers frequently experience an acute illness 3-8 weeks after infection, associated with egg deposition by adult worms. Diagnosis requires microscopic analysis of urine and stool. The disease is usually mild in travelers, since major symptoms, associated with high worm burdens, only occur after repeated exposure. Testing is usually delayed until after travel is complete. When traveling in endemic areas swimming and other contacts with fresh water should be avoided.

Other liver flukes may be acquired in Asia by eating raw, poorly cooked, smoked, or pickled freshwater fish. Infection is usually asymptomatic and diagnosed as an incidental finding during stool exam after travel to an endemic area.

Despite cholera being endemic in south Asia, the risk to travelers is generally low, unless working in a refugee camp, urban slum, or epidemic setting. Vaccination is not routinely recommended, but one should exercise care with food and water sources.

Rabies is endemic in south Asia, with up to 50% of Thai dogs testing positive. What's more, of those positive, 40% were puppies, when contact with humans is most common. Pre-exposure vaccination is recommended only for travelers with vocational exposure (ie. Veterinarians), children living in endemic areas, or travelers who will be in areas where dog rabies is common and where access to effective treatment after exposure is not available within a few days. This could include travelers "off the grid". The decision of whether to be vaccinated before travel depends on your itinerary and should be discussed with your personal physician. American consulates abroad can often provide information for travelers in need of POST EXPOSURE vaccination. Avoiding contact with dogs in these areas is clearly prudent.

The bacteria responsible for Plague exists in Myanmar and Vietnam. Since strategies to avoid mosquitos (due to Malaria risk) are also effective for the fleas that transmit plague, prudent travelers should be at very low risk. The illness presents with fever, chills, headache, weakness, and the appearance of swollen tender lymph nodes. If not treated, the bacteria may enter the bloodstream leading to pneumonia or meningitis. Treatment with Doxycycline or Ciprofloxacin is effective, reducing mortality to 10-20%. Plague pneumonia continues to have a 50% mortality rate even with treatment.

Although this sounds terrifying, one should bear in mind that plague is also endemic in the U.S. southwest and pacific coastal states, where chipmunks are the primary reservoir. About 100 cases of bubonic plague occur in the U.S.A. annually, yet we travel and camp in the involved areas. Exposure during travel in SE Asia would be greatest in rural villages. Protection against insects with an insect repellant containing 30% DEET is recommended.

Marine Risks include the neurotoxic jellyfish and blue-ringed octopus mentioned previously, as well as sea snakes and cone shells. Cone shells are beautiful predatory marine snails that are prized by collectors. The harpoon-like modified tooth loaded with poison in its proboscis is capable of penetrating gloves and wetsuits. When it senses prey, the harpoon is fired from the proboscis by a strong muscular contraction, injecting a neurotoxin that paralyzes its prey. Cone snails have a number of toxic harpoons that can fire in any direction, even backward. Large cones hunt and kill small fish, and their poison can be fatal to humans. Symptoms include intense pain, swelling, numbness, and tingling. Severe cases progress to muscle paralysis, vision changes, respiratory failure, and death. None of these organisms are aggressive. Humans become victims when they handle or threaten animals, so the best advice is: If you don't know what it is, don't touch it!

Sea Snakes are common around coral reefs in the Pacific and Indian oceans, most being from 3 to 6 feet in length. They live entirely at sea, having a flattened tail with which they can swim in either direction. Sea snake venom is highly toxic, but they are NOT aggressive. Bites are most common in local fishermen when removing them from their nets. Bites are initially asymptomatic.. Within 3 hours pain develops in muscles and joints, followed by paralysis, drooling, and blurred vision. A fatal outcome occurs in only 3% of documented bites. Treatment involves splinting and wrapping the extremity in an elastic bandage, which is loosened for 90 seconds every 10 minutes. If signs of envenomation occur, the child should be brought to local medical attention, as antivenin is available and effective. Avoidance is obviously advised.

<u>Africa</u>

Overland travel in Africa is most common in the southern and eastern subcontinent, where climate varies between temperate and tropical depending on elevation and latitude. In 1977 my wife and 5-year-old son joined me for an 8,000 km. overland camping trip, traveling from Botswana to Kenya and back. During this sojourn, we crossed deserts and dry savanna woodlands in Botswana, as well as rain forests and tropical jungles in Tanzania, Malawi, Mozambique, and Zimbabwe. We exercised precautions regarding mosquito and other arthropod vectors,

Avoid fresh water contact, and used prophylaxis for malaria. It was the trip of a lifetime and none of us experienced any significant illness. At the end of our three-year residence in southern Africa, we underwent screening for asymptomatic tropical and infectious diseases. None were found.

Malaria exists throughout Africa, but is usually seasonal and often limited to specific locales within countries. Reference should be made to the CDC website for recommendations for pro-phylaxis regarding your specific itinerary. Risk is also reduced by the use of permethrin-treated clothing, sleeping nets, and insect repellants containing DEET. These precautions also help avoid the insect vectors of other diseases transmitted by arthropods, including Dengue Fever, African sleeping sickness, plague, and rickettsial diseases. Avoiding untreated drinking water and uncooked foods reduces the risk of enteric fevers, diarrhea, and hepatitis A.

Swimming and bathing in bodies of freshwater carry the risk of Schistosomiasis in some areas. During our residence in Africa, a U.S.Peace Corps volunteer ignored the advice of local villagers swimming in a placid appearing river. He was killed by a crocodile. Another volunteer in north-ern Botswana failed to follow our advice and acquired schistosomiasis by bathing in a local stream. The risks of living and traveling in Africa are real. Although not entirely avoidable, they are manageable, if reasonable precautions are taken.

Infections such as Tuberculosis and River Blindness exist but require prolonged intimate exposure, not likely during travel. Other diseases such as rabies and schistosomiasis require only a brief contact for transmission but are easily avoided.

In Subsaharan west Africa (Nigeria, Mali, Burkina Faso, Chad, and Niger) meningococcal epidemics occur every 5-10 years. Travelers to these countries should consider being vaccinated with the meningococcal polysaccharide vaccine before departure.

Snake bites

Venomous snakebite in Africa is largely an occupational hazard for agricultural workers. Despite the presence of numerous cobras and mambas, large agile and highly venomous snakes, the majority of bites are due to small vipers and adders, which rely on camouflage for their survival. The big deadly snakes are alert, are not aggressive, and will flee from humans, if given the opportunity. Only when cornered, threatened, or stepped on are snakes likely to bite. Vipers are most active at night. Never walk through the bush without a light, and be careful where you step. Since leopards and lions feed at night, nocturnal sojourns on foot carry risks beyond snakes! Although I have tried to outline the health hazards of travel, one should not lose sight of its benefits, which greatly outweigh the risks. Prudent precautions can all but eliminate the risk of infectious diseases and envenomations. Careful preparation is warranted both in considering your itinerary and the medications to carry when "off the grid". That being said, the experience of a lifetime awaits those who leave the resorts behind and venture into the real world.

Appendix I

Drugs and dosages for children

By convention pediatric drug doses are calculated in mg. per KILOGRAM body weight. To convert your child's weight to kilograms, divide the weight in pounds by 2.2. For example a 44 lb. child's weight in kg. would be 44/2.2 = 20kg.

Recommended dosage forms for travelers are based on stability and ease of transport/storage. Where available tablets are suggested as they are easily transported, do not require refrigeration, and may be split and crushed. Capsules may be sprinkled on a small amount of food. Many pediatric formulations are available as powders that require mixing or dilution. These I have omitted as they are difficult to store and prone to mixing errors. If traveling by land, many drugs may be available thru local pharmacies. If at sea, your own supplies must suffice. Whether to rely on purchasing medications abroad or obtain them prior to departure requires consideration of the likelihood of their need and the difficulty of procurement based on your travel plans.

Acetaminophen (Tylenol): fever and mild pain

Recommended Dosage forms: solution or syrup 160mg/5ml

* oral disintegrating tablet 80mg and 160mg

* chewable tablet 80mg

Pediatric dosage: 10mg/kg given every 4-6 hours

Albuterol (xopenex)

Recommended dosage form: metered dose inhaler with spacer

Pediatric Dosage: 3-5 puffs every 15 minutes acutely and then every 4

hours until stable

Amoxicillin

Recommended Dosage Forms: *125 mg chewable tablet (may be crushed for young children)

*250 mg chewable tablet (may also be swallowed)

Pediatric dosage: 50mg/kg given twice daily for 10 days

Amoxicillin clavulanate (Augmentin)

Recommended Dosage form: 200mg and 400mg chewable tablet

Pediatric Dosage; Mild infection 20mg/kg/day divided twice daily

Severe infection: 40mg/kg/day divided twice daily

Atovaquone/proguanil

Recommended dosage forms: pediatric tablet: 62 mg atovaquone/25mg proquanil

adult tablet: 250 mg atovaquone/100mg proguanil

Pediatric dosage: Prophylaxis of Malaria

10-20 kg.: One pediatric tablet daily

20-20 kg.: Two pediatric tablets daily

30-40 kg.: Three pediatric tablets daily

Note: begin 1-2 days prior to entering malarious area and continue for 7 days after leaving area.

Treatment of uncomplicated Malaria: 10-20 kg.: one Adult tablet daily x 3 days

20-30 kg.: two Adult tablets daily x 3 days

30-40 kg.: three Adult tablets daily x 3 days

Azithromycin

Recommended Dosage Form: 250mg and 500mg tablets

Pediatric Dosage: Otitis/sinusitis: 10mg/kg/day once daily x 3 days

Pneumonia: 10mg/kg on day one, followed by 5mg/kg for 4 days

Typhoid fever: 10-20mg/kg daily for 7 days.

Bismuth subsalicylate (Pepto Bismol)

Recommended Dosage forms: 262mg chewable tablet

Pediatric dosage: every 1/2 hour for diarrhea. Maximum 8 doses/day

> 12 yr. 2 tablets

9-12yr. 1 tablet

6-9 yrs. 2/3 tablet

3-6 yr. 1/3 tablet (< 3 years - not recommended.)

Cefdinir (Omnicef)

Recommended dosage form: 300 mg capsule

Pediatric Dosage: 14 mg/kg/day given once daily

Cefixime (Suprax)

Recommended dosage form: 100 or 200mg chewable tablet

Pediatric Dosage: 16 mg/kg once daily on day on 8 mg/kg once daily 7-14 day

Cefpodoxime (Vantin)

Recommended Dosage forms: 100mg and 200mg tablets (may be

divided/crushed)

Pediatric Dosage: 5mg/kg/day divided twice daily

Cefprozil (Cefzil)

Recommended dosage form: 250 and 500 mg tablets

Pediatric Dosage: 15-30 mg/kg/day, divided twice daily

Ceftibuten (Cedax)

Recommended dosage form: 400 mg capsule

Pediatric Dosage: 9 mg/kg given once daily

Cefuroxime (Ceftin, Zinacef)

Recommended Dosage Forms: 250mg and 500mg tablets

Pediatric Dosage: 30mg/kg/day divided twice daily.

Chloramphenicol (not available in the U.S.)

Recommended Dosage Form: 250 mg capsule, open and mix with food.

Pediatric Dosage: for meningitis: 100 mg/kg/day divided every 6 hr.

Ciprofloxacin (Cipro) - not recommended for children due to degenerative joint disease in juvenile dogs, which has never been seen in humans.

Recommended Dosage form: 250mg tablet

Pediatric Dosage: 30mg/kg/day divided every 12 hr.

Ciprodex Otic Drops

Pediatric dosage: 4 drops in affected ear twice daily for 7 days.

Clindamycin (Cleocin)

Recommended dosage form: capsules of 75 and 150mg

Pediatric dosage: 20 mg/kg/day, divided every 6-8 hours

Dexamethasone

Recommended Dosage Forms: 2mg, 4mg, 6mg. table

Pediatric Dose: 0.6mg/kg once only, not to exceed 16mg.

Diphenhydramine (Benadryl)

Recommended Dosage form: 25mg and 50mg tablet

12.5mg chewable tablet

Pediatric Dosage: mild allergies: 5mg/kg/day divided every 6 hrs.

Anaphylaxis : 1-2mg/kg/dose

Doxycycline (generic)

Recommended Dosage Forms: tablets of 50, 75, 100mg.

Pediatric dose: < 45 kg., 2.2 mg/kg twice daily

> 45 kg., 100 mg twice daily

Malaria prophylaxis: 2.2 mg./kg once daily beginning 1-2 days before

travel and continuing for 4 weeks after leaving endemic area.

Malaria treatment: 2.2 mg/kg twice daily for 7 days combined with

quinine sulfate treatment.

Fluconazole for treatment of fungal infections

Recommended dosage form: 50 mg. or 100 mg. tablets

Pediatric dosage: 6 mg/kg. once weekly for 2-6 weeks

Griseofulvin (microsize) for fungal infections

Recommended dosage form: 125, 250 and 500 mg tablets

Pediatric Dosage: 20 - 25 mg/kg/day, given once daily

Hydroxyzine (Atarx, Vistaril)

Recommended dosage form: 10mg, 25mg and 50mg tablets

Pediatric Dosage: 2 mg/kg/day divided every 6-8 hrs.

Itraconazole for fungal infections

Recommended dosage form: capsule 100 mg.

Pediatric dosage: 3-5 mg/kg per day for one week

Mefloquine

Recommended dosage form: 250 mg tablet

Pediatric Dosage: for prophylaxis of Malaria

10-20 kg.: 1/4 tablet each week

20-30 kg.: 1/2 tablet each week

30-40 kg.: 3/4 tablet each week

Note: begin two weeks prior to entry into malarious area and continue for 4 weeks after leaving area. May cause vomiting. Administer with food or ample water.

Midazolam (Versed)

Recommended dosage form: syrup 2mg/ml

Pediatric dosage: .25 - .5 mg/kg given once only. Maximum 20mg.

Ondansetron (Zofran): vomiting

Recommended Dosage forms: 4 and 8mg oral dissolving tablet

Pediatric dosage: > 6 mo. of age: .15mg/kg/4-8 hrs.

4-12 yrs.: 8gm every 12 hrs.

Prednisone

Recommended dosage form: 10mg 15mg and 30mg orally disintegrating tablets

Pediatric dosage: 1-2mg/kg/day divided twice daily for 5 days

Quinine sulfate

Recommended dosage form: 324 mg or 200 mg capsule

Pediatric dosage: treatment of Malaria: 10 mg/kg/dose given every 8 hours for 3-7 days.

Note: use with doxycycline twice daily for 7 days.

Phenazopyridine (Pyridium) for symptoms of cystitis

Recommended dosage form: 100 mg tablet.

Pediatric dosage: < 12 years of age 4 mg/kg every 8 hours

> 12 years of age 200 mg every 8 hours

Terbinafine treatment of fungal skin infections

Recommended dosage form: 250 mg. Tablet

Pediatric dosage: 10-20 kg.: 62.5 mg daily for 2 weeks

20-40 kg.: 125 mg daily for 2 weeks

over 40 kg. : 250 mg. daily for 2 weeks

Appendix II

Information sources for international health

wwwnc.cdc.gov/travel/diseases

www.searo.who.int/en/

www.medscape.com

www.uptodate.com

The International Traveler's Guide to Avoiding Infections Charles E. Davis, M.D. ,Johns Hopkins University Press, 2012.

Appendix III

International medical evacuation insurance

airmedcarenetwork.com

globalrescue.com

Internationalsos.com

medjetassist.com

diversalertnetwork.com (covers sailors)

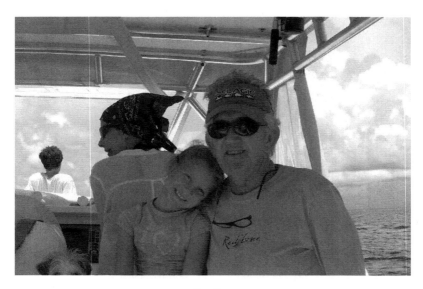

Caption

Authors Bio:

After his internship, Dr. LaGrone joined the US Peace Corps in Botswana and traveled throughout southern Africa with his family. After his pediatric residency, he moved to Pago Pago, American Samoa, where he served as Chief of Pediatrics at the LBJ Tropical Medical Center. The LaGrones then traveled overland through Java, Bali, and New Guinea, before sailing 7,500 miles across the Indian Ocean to Africa. For 25 years he practiced as a board-certified Pediatrician in Mississippi, taking time for medical relief missions in response to Haiti's earthquake and cholera epidemic and to the Philippines after super typhoon Haiyan. During the last decade, he has captained his sailboat throughout the Caribbean. His advice on the intersection of foreign travel and children's health should relieve your anxiety if considering travels "off the grid" as a family.